AIR FRYER LOW CARB COOKBOOK FOR DIABETICS

Healthy And Delicious Recipes for Preventing Or Reversing Diabetes

Diabetes Meal Plan For Beginners

Book 1

BY
NATALIE CHAMBERS

TABLE OF CONTENTS

INTRODUCTION

As a thank you for purchasing this book, I have compiled a list of 12 frequently asked questions about diabetes. Kindly email **RealNatalieChambers@gmail.com** to collect your bonus.

This book contains valuable information regarding diabetes, what it is, the warning signs, and different types, as well as, the sort of food diabetics can eat.

Diabetes is a kind of disease that occurs when your blood glucose is too high. This glucose serves as your chief source of energy, which generally comes from food. The insulin aids the glucose coming from food to get into your cells for energy. There are times when the body fails to generate enough insulin. As a result, glucose remains in the blood without getting through your cells.

In due course, there have been too much glucose found in the blood and this could cause serious health problems. Diabetes has no cure. But with the right knowledge and immediate prevention, it would be easier to manage or hopefully reverse the warning signs.

Also called as borderline diabetes or touch of sugar, these coined terms are meant for those who don't really have full blown diabetes, but either way, having one is a serious case.

There are different types of diabetes: type 1, type 2, and gestational diabetes.

Type 1 diabetes

Type 1 diabetes means that the body does not make insulin. It is like your body has rage war on your immune system, attacks, and damages the cells in the pancreas, which is the primary organ that makes insulin. Type 1 diabetes can appear at any age you are in. Even children can be diagnosed with type 1 diabetes. If you have one, this means that you have to take insulin on a daily basis in order to survive.

Type 2 diabetes

Type 2 diabetes is the most common type and is often called as lifestyle diabetes. Although this type of diabetes knows no age, it most often occur during middle age and latter age of life.

Gestational diabetes

This is a type of diabetes that occurs during pregnancy. More often than not, this disappears once the child is born. However, take note that when you develop gestational diabetes when you were pregnant, you have a higher chance of acquiring type 2 diabetes. In most cases, gestational diabetes actually means type 2 diabetes.

Symptoms of diabetes:

- intensified hunger
- blurry vision
- inexplicable weight loss
- exhaustion and low energy
- increased thirst and urination
- numbness in the hands or feet
- wounds that do not heal

Type 1 diabetes' symptoms can start instantly. It could be in a matter of days or weeks. On the other hand, type 2 diabetes develop gradually and could take several years. It is so slow that you won't even notice that you already have one. Many people who already have type 2 diabetes said that there are really no symptoms on the onset. In fact, they are unable to diagnose it until a diabetes-related issue starts to surface such as hypertension, heart problems, and even blurry vision.

This book will likewise shed light on how important it is to follow a low carb diet as well as the many recipes that you can create adhering to said diet.

Thanks for downloading this book, I hope you enjoy it!

CHAPTER 1 - DIABETES NUTRITION

Why is Nutrition Important for Diabetics?

Diabetes and proper nutrition should go hand in hand to help control your blood sugar level, weight, and ward off diabetes-related diseases. A diabetes diet means eating healthy, low carb food. It also means sticking to your portions and keeping everything moderate.

A diabetes diet is a kind of eating plan that's low in calories and carbs, but is rich in nutrients. The key elements here are vegetables, low carb fruits, and whole grains. In point of fact, a diabetes diet is considered to be the best diet regimen for almost everyone.

Nutrition is important for people with diabetes because it is the only way that you can delay the complications of diabetes and have it become full blown. This is why a healthy eating plan is always suggested to patients who have borderline diabetes.

When you eat too many carbs and calories that are way beyond the daily recommended amount, the glucose level becomes extremely high. When this happens, it could lead to hyperglycemia or high blood glucose level. If this persists, it could possibly lead to serious heart and kidney damage.

By adhering to a healthy meal plan, you can lower the level of your blood glucose. For those who have type 2 diabetes, the best way to control glucose level is through weight loss.

Creating a Meal Plan

To create a diabetes, low carb diet, you may incorporate different approaches to keep your blood glucose level at a safe range. Check out the following methods and choose which one works for you:

1. Counting carbohydrates

Carbohydrates is deemed to have a great influence in the level of your blood glucose. This, when broken down, turn into glucose. To help control it, you must learn how to compute your carbohydrates consumed for the day. This helps not just in limiting your portions, but also in adjusting the dosage of your insulin.

A dietician can help you in this and will educate you on how to read labels and measure your food. You will also be taught about the carb content of each food item as well as the right serving size.

2. The Plate Method

The ADA or American Diabetes Association suggests an easy way to your meals. It mainly highlights the consumption of more vegetables. As you prep your plate, this guideline must be followed:

- Half of your plate must be filled with non-starchy vegetables. This often includes carrots, spinach, and tomatoes.
- A quarter of your plate must be filled with protein. This can be chicken, fish, or lean pork.
- The last quarter must be filled with whole-grain item like starchy vegetables, brown rice, or green peas.
- It would also be good if you will try to incorporate small amounts of good fats such as chopped avocadoes and nuts.
- For your drink, you can add up unsweetened coffee, tea, milk, or fresh fruit juice.

When you ask for the help of a dietitian, they could teach you how food portions are measured and how labels are read. You will also learn that serving size and plate portioning play a major role in sticking to your diet.

3. Choose your food

Choose specific food to make meal planning easier. Choose the ones that are low carb and try to categorize each like carbs, protein, and fats. Each serving will be called "choice" that contains the same amount of proteins, carbs, and fat. This will have similar effect to your blood glucose as every other food of similar category.

How to Read Food Labels

When you go on a diabetic diet or just about any kind of diet, it is vital that you understand and know how to read labels. Getting a good grip of what's in your food is the secret to stocking good and nutritious food in the pantry. However, things get complicated when we encounter terms such as no additives, natural, and fresh. They tend to be confusing not because you don't know the meaning of these terms, it's because you don't really know which ones better and those that are just for show.

The following are essential information that you need to look into:

Calories. The first thing you need to look for when reading labels are the calories per serving as this count for weight control. The FDA has made calorie counting easier by placing it in labels of food appear larger and in bolder form.

Next thing is to look for the number of servings and serving size per container. This information is crucial to knowing the whole thing on the label.

Fat. It has more calories per gram than protein or carbs, and all fats contain 9 calories per gram. Limit food with trans and saturated fats and choose unsaturated fats whenever possible. In 2006, food manufacturers were instructed to list the quantity of trans fat per serving. Meanwhile, search for terms such as hydrogenated or partially hydrogenated indicating that the product has trans fats.

Dietary Fiber. This satisfies you and helps you become fuller longer. Your daily recommended dietary fiber is 25 grams every day. To be called high in fiber, your food must contain fiber of at least 5 grams per serving. Some examples include whole grain fiber, fruits, and vegetables.

Sugar. When you look at the labels, you will see terms such as dextrose, high fructose corn syrup, turbinado, and invert sugar among others. When you see this, they only mean sugar. Now, to choose wisely, go for at least 5 grams of any of these per serving to control your calories intake.

Sodium. In a day, sodium intake must be limited to 2,300 mg. This equates to less than 1 teaspoon for healthy adults and 1,500 mg for those who have health issues or those with family background of high blood pressure. If you want to decrease your sodium intake, choose food with reduced sodium.

% DV or % Daily Value. This is the fraction of a specific nutrient based on a 2,000 calorie diet. This provides you with an estimate of the nutrient contribution to one's diet. The nutrients emphasized in the % Daily Value are just a fractional list.

Ingredient List. All food manufacturers are required to record all ingredients included in a food merchandise by weight, and arrange them from the main ingredient down to the least amount of ingredient. So, if you're going to buy a jar of olives, the first ingredient list is the olives, of course. This lets you know that it is the main ingredient. The herb or spice listed on the last part of the ingredients' list contains the least amount. Those people with allergies or who are conscious about their weight can benefit greatly in reading the ingredients' list first.

The Food and Drug Administration has set detailed rules for what food producers can call reduced, low, light, and free, and other food nutritional jargons. The following are the terms to watch out for:

✓ When you see the word "healthy" in the label, this food should mean in layman's term that is limited in sodium, cholesterol, and low in fats.

✓ "Low cholesterol" food in the label may contain 2 grams of saturated fat and a maximum cholesterol of 20 milligrams.

✓ Food labeled "low sodium" may have a limit amount of 140 milligrams per serving.

✓ Organic food labels found in each pack of food are not necessarily healthy.

✓ Anything that is labeled "free" must only contain small quantities of ingredient per serving. Take for instance, food labeled as fat free or trans fat free can only have 0.5 mg of fat or trans fats.

✓ Food labeled "cholesterol-free" may only have 2 grams of saturated fat and 2 milligrams cholesterol.

✓ One serving of food labeled as "low-calorie" may have 40 calories maximum amount.

✓ One serving of food labeled as "low-fat" may have 3 grams fat maximum.

✓ One serving of food labeled as "reduced" ought to have 25% reduced amount of the ingredient than the regular version.

✓ One serving of food labeled as "light" ought to have 50% reduced amount of fat or calories than the regular version.

Recommended Daily Carb Intake for Diabetics

Understanding how many carbs you are allowed to eat on a daily basis if you are diabetic can be downright confusing. According to dietary guidelines, it is recommended that you go around between 45 to 60 percent of your daily caloric needs from carbohydrates if you are diabetic. But, there's also a growing number of studies from the medical experts that you eat fewer carbs or at least half of said percentage.

Ketogenic or very low-carb diet

A diet that is comprised of very low carb naturally encourage slight to moderate ketosis. This is a state where the body make use of fat and ketones instead of sugar as a main source of energy.

Ketosis happens when you consume fewer amount of carbs than 30-50 grams. This translates to no more than 2,000 calories. This has been prescribed to people with diabetes because it can significantly decrease the blood sugar levels that will help improve your heart health and promote weight loss.

Low-carb diets

A lot of low-carb diets limit carbs to 10 to 20% calories or 50 to 100 grams on a daily basis. Those who have type 1 diabetes and restrict the amount of carbs to 70 grams in a day have a tendency of a huge drop in their HbA1c from 7.7% to 6.4%. Their HbA1c levels also remained the same for a few years. This said reduction is very helpful in maintaining your blood sugar levels and in delaying the warning signs of diabetes.

Moderate-carb diet

This provides 20 to 35% calories or 100 to 150 grams of digestible carbohydrates on a daily basis. Doing this kind of diet can yield positive results to people with diabetes.

How to Find the Right Range

Based on research and scientific experiments, a low-carb restriction really does great wonders in lowering blood sugar levels. Since too much consumption of carbs could raise the blood sugar, significantly reducing them can assist in regulating the levels.

Take for example, if you are currently taking in an approximate amount of 250 grams of carbs every day, a reduction to 150 grams should result in lowering blood sugar after your meals. This being said, a restricted consumption of 20 to 50 grams seem to produce impressive outcomes, going so far as eliminating the need for diabetes maintenance or insulin medication.

The daily amount of carbohydrate, fat, and protein for diabetics vary from person to person. 1 gram of carb gives 4 calories. In order to get the number of carbs, you have to divide the number of calories from carbs. For instance, if you're going to eat 1,800 total of calories every day, your goal is to get at least 200 grams of carbs if you're going to consume 45 percent of calories from carbs.

You'll need to divide up out your carbohydrate intake throughout the day. A dietitian can help you know what food to eat, how much to eat, and when to eat based on your weight, activity level, medicines, and blood glucose targets.

Best Choices of Food for Diabetic People

Protein

- ✓ Canned tuna
- ✓ Salmon
- ✓ Lean pork
- ✓ Lean beef
- ✓ turkey, skinless
- ✓ chicken, skinless
- ✓ Eggs

- ✓ legumes
- ✓ Beans
- ✓ Greek yogurt, plain, nonfat
- ✓ unsalted nuts such as walnuts and almonds (eat in moderation)

Grains

- ✓ Quinoa
- ✓ Wild or brown rice
- ✓ Whole-wheat pasta
- ✓ Whole-grain breads
- ✓ Whole-grain cereal

Dairy

- ✓ Reduced-fat cheese (in moderation)
- ✓ Skim milk
- ✓ Nonfat, low-sodium cottage cheese
- ✓ Nonfat, unsweetened kefir

Non-starchy vegetables

- ✓ Cucumbers
- ✓ Jicama
- ✓ Cauliflower
- ✓ Spinach
- ✓ Onions
- ✓ Broccoli
- ✓ Brussels sprouts
- ✓ Kale
- ✓ Artichoke hearts Asparagus
- ✓ Swiss chard
- ✓ Peppers
- ✓ Baby Corn

Fruits

- ✓ Apples
- ✓ Oranges
- ✓ Peaches

- ✓ Pears
- ✓ Cherries
- ✓ Raspberries
- ✓ Blueberries
- ✓ Strawberries
- ✓ Melon
- ✓ Apricots
- ✓ Kiwi
- ✓ Bananas
- ✓ Grapes

Good fats

- ✓ Edamame
- ✓ Nut butters
- ✓ Avocados
- ✓ Nuts such as like pecans and pistachios
- ✓ Olives
- ✓ sunflower oil
- ✓ olive oil
- ✓ soybean oil
- ✓ corn oil
- ✓ chia seed
- ✓ flaxseed
- ✓ tuna
- ✓ salmon
- ✓ Tofu

List of Food to Avoid

Protein

- ❖ bologna
- ❖ Hotdogs
- ❖ Bacon
- ❖ Flavored or sweetened nuts
- ❖ Turkey
- ❖ Salami
- ❖ Ham

❖ Pepperoni
❖ Sweetened smoothies or Protein shakes
❖ Sausages
❖ Beef jerky

Grains

❖ White rice
❖ Pastries
❖ White bread
❖ Cereals
❖ White pasta

Dairy

❖ Reduced-fat or Full-fat milk
❖ Full-fat yogurt
❖ Reduced-fat or Full-fat cottage cheese
❖ Full-fat kefir, sweetened
❖ Full-fat cheese

Vegetables

❖ White potatoes
❖ Yams
❖ Corn
❖ Beets

Fruits

❖ Packaged juices
❖ Canned fruit in syrup
❖ Dried fruit
❖ Fresh juices

Bad fats

❖ palm oil
❖ Fast food
❖ Processed sweets

❖ Full-fat dairy products

❖ Packaged snacks

I hope what you've learned so far has been useful. If so, please can you spare 20 seconds to leave a review on Amazon letting me know what you think? I really appreciate

CHAPTER 2 – THE IMPORTANCE OF A LOW CARB DIET AND HOW IT CAN HELP DIABETICS

The Low Carb Diet

The low carb diet is essentially a kind of diet that limits carbohydrate intake from 50 to 150 grams per day. This literally means cutting down carb intake by at least 50 grams or more. Studies have proven that going on a low carb diet is beneficial for people who wanted to lose those extra pounds. This diet approach is proven effective weigh against other moderate meal plan diet.

The low carb diet gives emphasis on fat and protein. It likewise stimulates the body to use fat as fuel source instead of burning carbohydrates. If you wanted to improve your eating habits or prevent serious medical conditions such as high blood pressure, diabetes, metabolic disorder, and cardiovascular disease, the low carb diet is the way to go. Having a low carb diet also has a positive effect on improving your blood sugar levels.

How Does the Low Carb Diet Work?

Going through a low carb diet helps in decreasing the insulin levels in the blood. Insulin is the hormone that controls fat production and storage and blood sugar levels. Going low carb urges the body to use glucose more of an energy source rather than fat because fats are stored in the body when not used. Remember, decreased insulin levels could pave the way in burning more fat and use as fuel source. When this happens, food craving is reduced to a minimum.

Food that are deemed low in carbohydrates are rich in proteins. And protein is said to decrease hunger and helps stimulates metabolism. However, you must also be aware of the food that you will consume as some do not contain much nutrition so you'll only end up gaining more weight. The low carb diet eliminates these kinds of food and only encourages those that are loaded with essentials vitamins and minerals needed to stay healthy.

The Advantages of a Low Carb Diet for Diabetics

- ✓ It helps maintain low blood sugar level
- ✓ This diet is low in sugar and abundant in protein
- ✓ You still get to eat delicious and healthy eats

✓ It curbs appetite because the diet is rich in protein

The Challenges of a Low Carb Diet for Diabetics

❖ Limits your fruit intake especially those that are high in sugar
❖ Unhealthy fats and the risk of having higher LDL cholesterol
❖ Expect to have meals that are low in fiber and antioxidants.

While going low carb is advantageous, it is feared that this diet can be harmful to your health if practiced long term. Since you are deprived of nutrients, this diet will often leave you low on energy. To put in perspective, this diet can yield positive weight loss results, but expect to miss out on important nutrients especially the digestive challenges of eating food that are low in fiber. This paves the way for the balance of nutrient composition to be lost.

Bottom Line

Choosing a low carb diet would mean having to follow a structured meal plan whilst making exercise a part of your daily regimen. Also, it is important to count calories. Ignoring calorie limits would only make you gain weight even if you are eating low carb. The same concept as with any other forms of diet regimen - no matter how healthy your meal plan is - if you consume more food than what you burn, your weight loss goals will still fall to the hard shoulder. And so, despite efforts of losing all the inches and pounds, you still feel stuck.

Therefore, it is advised that you take a moment to listen to your body cues. It is still important that you go for a kind of diet that works best for your body – either low carb, low calorie, or low fat. Do not forget to find your balance. As you cut on carbohydrates, still find pleasure in eating good carbs such as vegetables, fruits, whole grains, and some dairy alternatives.

CHAPTER 3 - BREAKFAST RECIPES

AIR FRYER MEATBALLS IN TOMATO SAUCE

NUTRITION FACTS:

Calorie: 129
Carbohydrate: 15.4g
Fat: 17.8g
Protein: 17.6g
Fiber: 1.2g

Prep. Time: 10 minutes
Serves: 3-4

INGREDIENTS:

- 1 egg
- 3/4 pound lean ground beef
- 1 onion, chopped
- 3 tablespoons breadcrumbs
- 1/2 tablespoon fresh thyme leaves, chopped
- ½ cup tomato sauce
- 1 tablespoon parsley, chopped
- Pinch of salt
- Pinch of pepper, to taste

INSTRUCTIONS:

1. Preheat the Air Fryer to 390 degrees
2. Place all ingredients in a bowl. Mix until well-combined. Divide mixture into 12 balls. Place in the cooking basket.
3. Cook meatballs for 8 minutes.
4. Put the cooked meatballs in an oven dish. Pour the tomato sauce on top. Put the oven dish inside the cooking basket of the Air Fryer.
5. Cook for 5 minutes at 330 degrees.

CHICKEN FRIED SPRING ROLLS

NUTRITION FACTS:

Calorie: 150

Carbohydrate: 18g

Fat: 5g

Protein: 9g

Fiber: 1.5g

Prep. Time: 20 minutes

Serves: 4

INGREDIENTS

For the spring roll wrappers

- 1 egg, beaten
- 8 spring roll wrappers
- 1 teaspoon cornstarch
- 1/2 teaspoon olive oil

FOR THE FILLING

- 1 cup chicken breast, cooked, shredded
- 1 celery stalk, sliced thinly
- 1 carrot, sliced thinly
- 1 teaspoon chicken stock powder, low sodium
- 1/2 teaspoon ginger, chopped finely
- 1/2 cup of sliced mushrooms

INSTRUCTIONS:

1. Preheat the Air Fryer to 390 degrees.
2. Prepare the filling. In a bowl, combine shredded chicken, mushrooms, carrot, and celery. Add in chicken stock powder, and ginger. Stir well.
3. Meanwhile, mix cornstarch and egg until thick in a bowl. Set aside.
4. Spoon some filling into a spring roll wrapper. Roll and seal the ends with the egg mixture.
5. Lightly brush spring rolls with oil and place them in the cooking basket. Cook for 4 minutes. Serve.

MUSHROOM AND CHEESE FRITTATA

NUTRITION FACTS:

Calorie: 140

Carbohydrate: 5.4g

Fat: 10.6g

Protein: 22.7g

Fiber: 1.2g

Prep. Time: 20 minutes

Serves: 4

INGREDIENTS

- 6 eggs
- 6 cups button mushrooms, sliced thinly
- 1 red onion, sliced into thin rounds
- 6 tbsps. feta cheese, reduced fat, crumbled
- Pinch of salt
- 2 tbsps. olive oil

INSTRUCTIONS:

1. Preheat Air Fryer to 330 degrees F.
2. Saute onions and mushrooms. Transfer to a plate with paper towel.
3. Meanwhile, beat the eggs in a bowl. Season with salt. Coat a baking dish with cooking spray. Pour egg mixture.
4. Add in mushroom and onions. Top with crumbled feta cheese.
5. Place baking dish in the Airfryer basket. Cook for 20 minutes. Serve.

CINNAMON AND CHEESE PANCAKE

NUTRITION FACTS:

Calorie: 140

Carbohydrate: 5.4g

Fat: 10.6g

Protein: 22.7g

Fiber: 1.2g

Prep. Time: 5-7 minutes

Serves: 4

INGREDIENTS:

- 2 eggs
- 2 cups of cream cheese, reduced fat
- ½ teaspoon of cinnamon
- 1 pack Stevia

INSTRUCTIONS:

1. Preheat Air Fryer to 330 degrees F.
2. Meanwhile, combine cream cheese, cinnamon, eggs, and stevia in a blender.
3. Pour ¼ of the mixture in the Airfryer basket. Cook for 2 minutes on each side. Repeat the process with the rest of the mixture. Serve.

LOW-CARB WHITE EGG AND SPINACH FRITTATA

NUTRITION FACTS:

Calorie: 120
Carbohydrate: 13g
Fat: 4.5g
Protein: 9.9g
Fiber: 1.2g

Prep. Time: 12-15 minutes
Serves: 4

INGREDIENTS:

- 8 egg whites
- 2 cups of fresh spinach
- 2 tablespoons olive oil
- 1 green pepper, chopped
- 1 red pepper, chopped
- ½ cup of feta cheese, reduced fat, crumbled
- ¼ of a yellow onion, chopped
- 1 teaspoon salt
- 1 teaspoon pepper

INSTRUCTIONS:

1. Preheat the Air Fryer to 330 degrees F.
2. Meanwhile, place red and green peppers, and onions in the Air Fryer basket and cook for 3 minutes. Season with salt and pepper.
3. Pour egg whites and cook for 4 minutes. Add in the spinach and feta cheese on top.
4. Cook for 5 minutes.
5. Transfer to a plate. Slice and serve.

SCALLION SANDWICH

NUTRITION FACTS:

Calorie: 154

Carbohydrate: 9g

Fat: 2.5g

Protein: 8.6g

Fiber: 2.4g

Prep. Time: 10 minutes

Serves: 1

INGREDIENTS:

- 2 slices wheat bread
- 2 teaspoons butter, low fat
- 2 scallions, sliced thinly
- 1 tablespoon of parmesan cheese, grated
- 3/4 cup of cheddar cheese, reduced fat, grated

Instructions:

1. Preheat the Air fryer to 356 degrees.
2. Spread butter on a slice of bread. Place inside the cooking basket with the butter side facing down.
3. Place cheese and scallions on top. Spread the rest of the butter on the other slice of bread Put it on top of the sandwich and sprinkle with parmesan cheese.
4. Cook for 10 minutes.

LEAN LAMB AND TURKEY MEATBALLS WITH YOGURT

NUTRITION FACTS:

Calorie: 154

Carbohydrate: 9g

Fat: 2.5g

Protein: 8.6g

Fiber: 2.4g

Prep. Time: 10 minutes

Serves: 4

INGREDIENTS:

- 1 egg white
- 4 ounces ground lean turkey
- 1 pound of ground lean lamb
- 1 teaspoon each of cayenne pepper, ground coriander, red chili paste, salt, and ground cumin
- 2 garlic cloves, minced
- 1 1/2 tablespoons parsley, chopped
- 1 tablespoon mint, chopped
- 1/4 cup of olive oil

FOR THE YOGURT

- 2 tablespoons of buttermilk
- 1 garlic clove, minced
- 1/4 cup mint, chopped
- 1/2 cup of Greek yogurt, non-fat
- Salt to taste

INSTRUCTIONS:

1. Set the Air Fryer to 390 degrees.
2. Mix all the ingredients for the meatballs in a bowl. Roll and mold them into golf-size round pieces. Arrange in the cooking basket. cook for 8 minutes.
3. While waiting, combine all the ingredients for the mint yogurt in a bowl. Mix well.
4. Serve the meatballs with the mint yogurt. Top with olives and fresh mint.

AIR FRIED EGGS

NUTRITION FACTS:

Calorie: 106

Carbohydrate: 10g

Fat: 3.2g

Protein: 9.0g

Fiber: 1.2g

Prep. Time: 15 minutes

Serves: 4

INGREDIENTS:

- 4 eggs
- 2 cups of baby spinach, rinsed
- 1 tablespoon of extra-virgin olive oil
- 1/2 cup of cheddar cheese, reduced fat, shredded, divided
- Pinch of salt
- Pinch of pepper

INSTRUCTIONS:

1. Preheat the Air Fryer to 350 degrees.
2. Heat oil in a pan over medium-high flame. Cook the spinach until wilted. Drain the excess liquid. Put the cooked spinach into 4 greased ramekins.
3. Add a slice of bacon to each ramekin, crack an egg and put cheese on top. Season with salt and pepper.
4. Put the ramekins inside the cooking basket of the Air Fryer.
5. Cook for 15 minutes.

CINNAMON PANCAKE

NUTRITION FACTS:

Calorie: 106
Carbohydrate: 10g
Fat: 3.2g
Protein: 9.0g
Fiber: 1.2g

Prep. Time: 15 minutes
Serves: 4

INGREDIENTS:

- 2 eggs
- 2 cups of cream cheese, reduced fat
- ½ teaspoon cinnamon
- 1 pack Stevia

INSTRUCTIONS

1. Preheat Air Fryer to 330 degrees F.
2. Combine cream cheese, cinnamon, eggs, and stevia in a blender.
3. Pour ¼ of the mixture in the Airfryer basket.
4. Cook for 2 minutes on each side.
5. Repeat the process with the rest of the mixture. Serve.

SPINACH AND MUSHROOMS OMELET

NUTRITION FACTS:

Calorie: 110

Carbohydrate: 9g

Fat: 1.3g

Protein: 5.4g

Fiber: 1.0g

Prep. Time: 15 minutes

Serves: 4

INGREDIENTS:

- ½ cup spinach leaves
- 1 cup mushrooms
- 3 green onions
- 1 cup water
- ½ teaspoon turmeric
- 1/2 red bell pepper
- 2 tablespoons butter, low fat
- 1 cup of almond flour
- ½ teaspoon onion powder
- ½ teaspoon garlic powder
- ½ teaspoon fresh ground black pepper
- ¼ teaspoon ground thyme
- 2 tablespoons extra virgin olive oil
- 1 teaspoon black salt
- Salsa, store-bought

INSTRUCTIONS:

1. Preheat the Air Fryer to 300 degrees.
2. Rinse spinach leaves over tap water. Set aside.
3. In a mixing bowl, combine green onions, onion powder, garlic powder, red bell pepper, mushrooms, turmeric, thyme, olive oil, salt, and pepper. Mix well.
4. In another bowl, combine water and flour to form a smooth paste.

5. In a pan, heat olive oil. Saute peppers and mushrooms for 3 minutes. Tip in spinach and cook for 3 minutes. Set aside.

6. In the Airfryer basket, pour omelet batter. Cook for 3 minutes before flipping. Place vegetables on top. Season with salt. Serve with salsa on the side.

ALL BERRIES PANCAKES

NUTRITION FACTS:

Calorie: 57

Carbohydrate: 14g

Fat: 0.3g

Protein: 0.7g

Fiber: 2.4g

Prep. Time: 15 minutes

Serves: 4

INGREDIENTS:

- ½ cup frozen blueberries, thawed
- ½ cup frozen cranberries, thawed
- 1 cup coconut milk
- 2 Tbsp. coconut oil, for greasing
- 2 Tbsp. stevia
- 1 cup whole wheat flour, finely milled
- 1 Tbsp. baking powder
- 1 tsp. vanilla extract
- ¼ tsp. salt

DIRECTIONS:

1. Preheat Air Fryer to 330 degrees F.
2. In a mixing bowl, combine coconut oil, coconut milk, flour, stevia, baking powder, vanilla extract and salt.
3. Gently fold in berries. Divide batter into equal portions. Pour into the Airfryer basket. Flip once the edges are set. Do not press down on pancakes.
4. Transfer to a plate. Sprinkle palm sugar. Serve.

CHAPTER 4 - AIR FRYER LUNCH MENUS

AIR FRIED AUBERGINE AND TOMATO

NUTRITION FACTS:

Calorie: 140.3
Carbohydrate: 26.6g
Fat: 3.4g
Protein: 4.2g
Fiber: 7.3g

Prep. Time: 10 minutes
Serves: 2

INGREDIENTS:

- 1 aubergine, sliced thickly into 4 disks
- 1 tomato, sliced into 2 thick disks
- 2 tsp. feta cheese, reduced fat
- 2 fresh basil leaves, minced
- 2 balls, small buffalo mozzarella, reduced fat, roughly torn
- Pinch of salt
- Pinch of black pepper

INSTRUCTIONS:

1. Preheat Air Fryer to 330 degrees F.
2. Spray small amount of oil into the Airfryer basket. Fry aubergine slices for 5 minutes or until golden brown on both sides. Transfer to a plate.
3. Fry tomato slices in batches for 5 minutes or until seared on both sides.
4. To serve, stack salad starting with an aubergine base, buffalo mozzarella, basil leaves, tomato slice, and ½ teaspoon feta cheese.
5. Top of with another slice of aubergine and ½ tsp feta cheese. Serve.

QUICK FRY CHICKEN WITH CAULIFLOWER AND WATER CHESTNUTS

NUTRITION FACTS:

Calorie: 220

Carbohydrate: 13.6g

Fat: 9g

Protein: 30.5g

Fiber: 3.8g

Prep. Time: 15 minutes

Serves: 2-3

INGREDIENTS:

For the quick fry

- 1½ pounds chicken thigh fillets, diced
- 1 piece, small red bell pepper, julienned
- 1 piece, thumb-sized ginger, grated
- 2 Tbsp. olive oil
- 1 clove, large garlic, minced
- 2 stalks, large leeks, minced
- 1 can, 5 oz. water chestnuts, quartered
- 1 head, small cauliflower, cut into bite-sized florets
- ¾ cups chicken stock, low sodium

SEASONINGS

- 1 tsp. stevia
- 1 Tbsp. fish sauce
- ½ Tbsp. cornstarch, dissolved in
- 4 Tbsp. water
- Pinch of salt
- Pinch of black pepper, to taste

GARNISH:

- leeks, minced
- 1 piece, large lime, cut into 6 wedges

DIRECTIONS:

1. Preheat Air Fryer to 330 degrees F.
2. Pour olive oil in a pan. Swirl pan to coat. Saute garlic, ginger, and leeks for 2 minutes. Set aside. Add in water chestnuts, cauliflower, red bell pepper, and chicken broth. Stir well. Cook for 15 minutes.
3. Meanwhile, put the chicken in the Airfryer basket. Fry until seared and golden brown.
4. Add in seasoning into the pan. Stir and cook until the juice thickens.
5. Ladle 1 portion of quick fry veggies and chicken, Garnish with leeks and lemon wedges on the side. Serve.

CHEESY SALMON FILLETS

NUTRITION FACTS:

Calorie: 274

Carbohydrate: 1g

Fat: 19g

Protein: 24g

Fiber: 0.5g

Prep. Time: 15 minutes

Serves: 2-3

INGREDIENTS:

For the salmon fillets

- 2 pieces, 4 oz. each salmon fillets, choose even cuts
- ½ cup sour cream, reduced fat
- ¼ cup cottage cheese, reduced fat
- ¼ cup Parmigiano-Reggiano cheese, freshly grated

GARNISH:

- Spanish paprika
- ½ piece lemon, cut into wedges

INSTRUCTIONS:

1. Preheat Air Fryer to 330 degrees F.
2. To make the salmon fillets, mix sour cream, cottage cheese, and Parmigiano-Reggiano cheese in a bowl.
3. Layer salmon fillets in the Airfryer basket. Fry for 20 minutes or until cheese turns golden brown.
4. To assemble, place a salmon fillet and sprinkle paprika. Garnish with lemon wedges and squeeze lemon juice on top. Serve.

TUNA STEAKS

NUTRITION FACTS:

Calorie: 120
Carbohydrate: 0g
Fat: 1g
Protein: 27g
Fiber: 0g

Prep. Time: 3-5 minutes
Serves: 1

INGREDIENTS:

For the tuna steaks

- 2 pieces bone-in tuna steaks
- Pinch of salt
- 1 Tbsp. olive oil

GARNISH:

- 1 Tbsp. homemade garlic and parsley butter, divided
- 2 Tbsp. toasted garlic flakes, divided
- ½ small lemon, cut into wedges

INSTRUCTIONS:

1. Preheat Air Fryer to 330 degrees F.
2. Season tuna steaks with salt.
3. Layer tuna inside the Air Fryer basket. Fry for 2 minutes on each side. Transfer on a plate.
4. To assemble, place steaks in each plate. Spread parsley and garlic butter. Serve with lemon wedges.

AIR-FRIED LEAN PORK TENDERLOIN

NUTRITION FACTS:

Calorie: 221

Carbohydrate: 8g

Fat: 10g

Protein: 22g

Fiber: 0g

Prep. Time: 5-7 minutes

Serves: 1

INGREDIENTS:

- 2 pork tenderloin, lean, sliced into matchsticks
- ½ red bell pepper, julienned
- ½ green bell pepper, julienned
- 1 white onion, sliced thinly
- 1 Tbsp. almond flour, finely milled
- 1 tsp. sea salt
- 1 tsp. ground black pepper
- ½ tsp. dried pepper flakes

INSTRUCTIONS:

1. Preheat Air Fryer to 330 degrees F.
2. Season pork tenderloin with salt, pepper, pepper flakes, and almond flour. Set aside.
3. Layer pork tenderloin in the Airfryer basket. Cook for 5 minutes or until golden brown.
4. Meanwhile, heat oil in a pan and stir fry onions and bell peppers for 1 minute.
5. To assemble, add cooked pork in a plate and put vegetables on the side. Serve.

AIR FRIED ARTICHOKE HEARTS

NUTRITION FACTS:

Calorie: 67

Carbohydrate: 7g

Fat: 3g

Protein: 2g

Fiber: 1g

Prep. Time: 5-7 minutes

Serves: 2-3

INGREDIENTS:

Artichokes

- 1 pound frozen artichoke hearts, thawed, quartered
- 1 cup plain yogurt, low fat
- 2 eggs, whisked
- 1 cup almond flour, finely milled
- 1 cup almond flour, coarsely milled
- 1 small lime, sliced into wedges, pips removed
- ½ cup sour cream, reduced fat
- Pinch of sea salt

INSTRUCTIONS:

1. Preheat Air Fryer to 330 degrees F.
2. In a bowl, combine yogurt and salt. Soak artichoke hearts for at 15 minutes. Drain. Discard yogurt.
3. Dredge artichokes in almond flour first, then into eggs, and into coarse-milled almond flour.
4. Layer artichoke hearts into the Air Fryer basket. Fry for 5 minutes or until golden brown on all sides. Drain on paper towels. Squeeze lime juice. Serve with lime wedges and sour cream on the side.

AIR-FRYER ONION STRINGS

NUTRITION FACTS:

Calorie: 150

Carbohydrate: 13g

Fat: 17g

Protein: 2g

Fiber: 1g

Prep. Time: 7-10 minutes

Serves: 3-4

INGREDIENTS:

- 2 cups buttermilk
- 1 piece, whole white onion, halved, julienned
- 2 cups almond flour, finely milled
- ½ tsp. cayenne pepper
- Pinch of sea salt
- Pinch of black pepper to taste

INSTRUCTIONS:

1. Preheat Air Fryer to 330 degrees F.
2. Soak onion strings in buttermilk for 1 hour before frying. Drain.
3. Meanwhile, mix almond flour, cayenne pepper, salt and pepper in a bowl. Coat onion strings with flour mixture.
4. Layer onions in Airfryer basket. Fry until golden brown and crisp. Drain on paper towels. Season with salt. Serve.

AIR FRIED SPINACH

NUTRITION FACTS:

Calorie: 81.6

Carbohydrate: 4.5g

Fat: 6.9g

Protein: 1.3g

Fiber: 1.1g

Prep. Time: 3-5 minutes

Serves: 3

INGREDIENTS:

- 2½ pounds fresh spinach leaves and tender stems only
- Pinch of sea salt, to taste

INSTRUCTIONS:

1. Preheat Air Fryer to 330 degrees F.
2. Put spinach in the Airfryer basket. Fry for 20 seconds. Drain on paper towels. Repeat step with the rest of the spinach. Season with salt. Serve.

AIR FRIED ZUCCHINI BLOOMS

NUTRITION FACTS:

Calorie: 117

Carbohydrate: 8g

Fat: 8g

Protein: 1g

Fiber: 0g

Prep. Time: 3-5 minutes

Serves: 3

INGREDIENTS:

- 2½ pounds zucchini flowers, rinsed
- 1 cup almond flour, finely milled
- Pinch of sea salt, to taste
- Balsamic vinegar, for garnish

DIRECTIONS:

1. Preheat Air Fryer to 330 degrees F.
2. Half-fill deep fryer with oil. Set this at medium heat. Lightly season zucchini flowers with salt, and then dredge in almond flour.
3. Layer breaded flowers into the Air Fryer basket Fry until golden brown. Drain on paper towels. Transfer to a plate. Pour balsamic vinegar if using. Serve.

CHAPTER 5 - DINNER SELECTIONS

AIR FRIED SALMON BELLY

NUTRITION FACTS:

Calorie: 129

Carbohydrate: 5.35g

Fat: 0.8g

Protein: 11.99g

Fiber: 0.3g

Prep. Time: 5-10 minutes

Serves: 2

INGREDIENTS:

Salmon belly

- 1 pound salmon belly, skin on, trimmed, sliced into ¾ inch thick sliver
- 2 Tbsp. almond flour, finely milled
- Pinch of sea salt

DIP

- ¼ tsp. fresh garlic, minced
- ½ cup coconut or palm vinegar
- ¼ cup white onion, minced
- ¼ tsp. fish sauce
- 1 piece bird's eye chili, deseeded, minced
- black pepper to taste

INSTRUCTIONS:

1. Preheat Air Fryer to 330 degrees F.
2. Combine palm vinegar, fish sauce, white onion, bird's eye chili, garlic, and pepper in a small bowl. Set aside.

3. Season salmon belly with the mixture. Roll in almond flour.
4. Layer fillet in the Air Fryer's basket. Fry for 5 minutes or until golden brown. Drain on paper towels.
5. Serve with dip or on bed of rice.

STUFFED PORTABELLA MUSHROOMS

NUTRITION FACTS:

Calorie: 129
Carbohydrate: 5.35g
Fat: 0.8g
Protein: 11.99g
Fiber: 0.3g

Prep. Time: 5-10 minutes
Serves: 2

INGREDIENTS:

- 2 dozen fresh portabella mushrooms, minced
- 2 tsp. olive oil, add more for drizzling/greasing

FILLING

- 1 Tbsp. olive oil
- 1 onion, minced
- 2 garlic cloves, grated
- 3 Tbsp. butter, unsalted
- ¼ cup apple cider vinegar
- 2 Tbsp. fresh parsley, minced
- ¼ cup roasted cashew nuts, crushed
- ¼ cup cheddar cheese, reduced fat, grated
- ¼ cup Parmesan cheese, grated
- Pinch of sea salt
- Pinch of black pepper to taste

INSTRUCTIONS:

1. Preheat Air Fryer to 330 degrees F.
2. Meanwhile, in a pan heat the oil. Saute onion and garlic for 2 minutes or until translucent and fragrant. Stir in butter, almonds, mushrooms stems, salt, and pepper. Cook for 3 minutes or until mushrooms turn brown in color.
3. Pour vinegar. Cook until the liquid is reduced. Stir in nuts and Parmesan cheese. Allow

mixture to cool.

4. Spoon mixture into mushroom caps. Layer mushrooms in the prepared baking dish. Place inside the Airfryer basket. Cook for 20 minutes. Serve.

BREADED LEAN PORK CHOPS ON SPINACH SALAD

NUTRITION FACTS:

Calorie: 165
Carbohydrate: 7.15g
Fat: 9.9g
Protein: 11.08g
Fiber: 0.5g

Prep. Time: 35-40minutes
Serves: 2

INGREDIENTS:

- 2 pieces lean pork chops, pounded ¼-inch thick using a meat mallet

BREADING AND SEASONINGS

- 1 egg, whisked
- ½ tsp. Dijon mustard
- ¼ tsp. dried oregano
- ½ cup almond flour, finely milled
- ¼ cup Parmesan cheese
- Pinch of sea salt
- Pinch of black pepper to taste

SALAD

- 6 cups baby spinach leaves, rinsed, spun-dried
- 2 Tbsp. apple cider vinegar
- 1 Tbsp. extra virgin olive oil
- Pinch of sea salt, to taste

INSTRUCTIONS:

- Preheat Air Fryer to 330 degrees F.
- In a bowl, mix egg, oregano, and mustard. Season with salt and pepper. Marinate pork chops for 30 minutes. Put inside the refrigerator before frying.

- In another bowl, mix almond flour and Parmesan cheese. Roll pork chops into breading.
- Layer pork chops in the Air Fryer basket for 5 minutes or until golden brown. Drain on paper towels.
- Put salad ingredients in a salad bowl. Put pork chop slivers. Mix well to combine. Serve.

PEPPERY BUTTER SWORDFISH STEAKS

NUTRITION FACTS:

Calorie: 140

Carbohydrate: 0g

Fat: 0g

Protein: 23g

Fiber: 0g

Prep. Time: 30 minutes

Serves: 4

INGREDIENTS:

Swordfish steaks and seasoning

- 4 pieces swordfish steaks, make shallow incisions through skin
- 1/16 tsp. salt
- 1 tsp. olive oil, for greasing

PEPPERY BUTTER

- 2 tsp. butter , unsalted
- ½ tsp. toasted garlic, store-bought
- 1 tsp. fresh parsley, minced
- ½ tsp. mixed dried ground peppercorns
- ½ lime, sliced into 4 equal wedges, for garnish

INSTRUCTIONS:

1. Preheat the Air Fryer to 400 degrees F.
2. Using a pastry brush, lightly grease four sheets of aluminum foil with olive oil. This will prevent steak from sticking to the foil, while preserving most of its juices.
3. Season swordfish steaks with salt. Wrap each piece individually in prepared sheets of aluminum foil.
4. Place two steaks into Air Fryer basket. Place double layer rack into the basket. Layer remaining fish on top.
5. Fry for 10 minutes. Shake contents of basket once midway through.
6. Remove steaks from machine. Place on a plate. Rest meat for 10 minutes before

removing aluminum foil sheets. Place swordfish steaks directly into plates, and drizzle in cooking juices.

7. Combine ingredients in a small microwave oven-safe bowl. Microwave for 3 seconds on highest heat until butter softens. Stir well.

8. Top each steak off with equal portions of peppery butter.

9. Squeeze lime juice over fish before eating.

AIR FRIED CITRUS BUTTER TILAPIA

NUTRITION FACTS:

Calorie: 189

Carbohydrate: 7g

Fat: 12g

Protein: 16g

Fiber: 0.6g

Prep. Time: 5-7 minutes

Serves: 2

INGREDIENTS:

- 2 large tilapia fillet
- 1 Tbsp. fresh cilantro, minced
- 2 tsp. sweet paprika powder
- 2 Tbsp. citrusy butter, unsalted
- 1 tsp. sea salt

INSTRUCTIONS:

1. Preheat the Air Fryer to 330 degrees F.
2. Season tilapia with salt and paprika. Set aside to drain in a colander.
3. Layer tilapia in the Airfryer basket. Fry fillets for 5 minutes or until crisp tender and brown all over.
4. Transfer cooked fillets on a plate. Pour citrusy butter. Garnish with cilantro. Serve.

LEAN PORK BELLY CRISP

NUTRITION FACTS:

Calorie: 145

Carbohydrate: 0g

Fat: 15g

Protein: 2g

Fiber: 0g

Prep. Time: 15 minutes

Serves: 2

INGREDIENTS:

- 2½ pounds lean pork belly, whole
- 2 dried bay leaves
- 2 tablespoons olive oil
- 2 Tbsp. fish sauce
- 2 cups vinegar
- 2 cups water
- 2 Tbsp. black peppercorns, lightly cracked

INSTRUCTIONS:

1. Preheat the Air Fryer to 330 degrees F.
2. Heat oil in the saucepan. Add pork belly, vinegar, water, fish sauce, bay leaves, and black peppercorns. Bring mixture to a boil.
3. Turn down heat to low. Allow to simmer for 10 minutes. Remove from heat. Drain pork in a colander.
4. Layer pork bell in the Air Fryer basket. Fry for 5 minutes or until golden brown. Serve with vegetable salad.

EASY BEEF CURRY WITH CARROTS AND CAULIFLOWER

NUTRITION FACTS:

Calorie: 209

Carbohydrate: 11g

Fat: 13g

Protein: 29g

Fiber: 2.9g

Prep. Time: 15 minutes

Serves: 2-4

INGREDIENTS

Beef curry and sauce

- 1 can thick coconut cream
- ¼ lean beef, sliced into sukiyaki strips
- ½ tsp. curry powder
- ½ tsp. garam masala
- ¼ tsp. ghee
- ⅛ tsp. fresh ginger, grated
- 1/16 tsp. fish sauce
- 1/16 tsp. salt
- 1/16 tsp. red pepper flakes
- 1/16 tsp. white pepper

- ¼ cup cauliflower, sliced into bite-sized florets
- ¼ cup shallots, peeled, diced
- 1 banana chili, stemmed, halved lengthwise, for garnish
- 1 cup fresh straw mushrooms, bases trimmed, halved lengthwise, rinsed, drained
- ¼ cup frozen baby peas, thawed, drained well

INSTRUCTIONS:

1. Preheat the Air Fryer to 355 degrees F.
2. Season beef with salt and pepper.
3. Combine remaining ingredients in a separate bowl.

4. Sprinkle veggies and mushrooms on top. Drape beef sukiyaki slices on top of veggies so these are partially covered. Leave some veggies exposed.

5. Pour in beef curry sauce. Seal lid.

6. Place filled tiffin box into Air Fryer basket. Cook dish for 5 minutes.

7. Turn down heat to 285 degrees F. Continue cooking for another 20 minutes. Turn off machine immediately. Leave tiffin box in the basket for 5 minutes to rest.

8. Remove tiffin box. Carefully take off lid. Garnish with banana chili. Serve right out of tiffin box.

MACKEREL STEAKS

NUTRITION FACTS:

Calorie: 220

Carbohydrate: 0g

Fat: 9.2g

Protein: 34.4g

Fiber: 0g

Prep. Time: 7-10 minutes

Serves: 2

INGREDIENTS:

- 2 pieces, 6 oz. each Spanish mackerel steaks
- 2 Tbsp. butter, unsalted, divided
- ¼ cup garlic, grated
- 2 Tbsp. olive oil
- Pinch of sea salt to taste

INSTRUCTIONS:

1. Preheat the Air Fryer to 330 degrees F.
2. Season mackerel steaks with salt.
3. Meanwhile, in a skillet, heat the oil. Saute garlic for 3 minutes or until limp and aromatic. Set aside.
4. Layer mackerel steaks in the Air Fryer basket. Fry got 4 minutes. Do not overcook. Transfer steaks to a plate. Drizzle in cooking liquid. Sprinkle garlic on top. Serve.

STIR-FRIED BROCCOLI STALKS

NUTRITION FACTS:

Calorie: 138

Carbohydrate: 0g

Fat: 1g

Protein: 19g

Fiber: 0g

Prep. Time: 3-5 minutes

Serves: 2

INGREDIENTS:

- 1 lb broccoli stalks, sliced into thin rounds
- ½ teaspoon olive brine
- ½ teaspoon caper brine
- Pinch dried chillies
- ½ teaspoon ground coriander
- ½ teaspoon ground cumin
- 3 black olives
- 2 garlic cloves, crushed
- Juice of 1 lemon
- ½ silver rind lemon
- 2 sun-dried tomatoes
- ½ tablespoons capers
- 3 cups stock
- Pinch of salt
- Pinch of pepper

INSTRUCTIONS:

1. Preheat the Air Fryer to 330 degrees F.
2. Combine garlic, onion, capers, chillies, olives, sun-dried tomatoes, olive and caper brines, cumin, coriander, lemon juice, lemon rind, and half the stock. Stir well. Bring mixture to a boil.
3. Meanwhile, layer broccoli stalks in the Airfryer basket. Fry for 2 minutes.
4. Wait for the mixture to become syrupy before adding the cooked broccoli stalks. Pour remaining lemon juice and stock. Season with salt and pepper. Serve.

CHAPTER 6 - AIR FRYER SNACKS

CHEESE STICKS

NUTRITION FACTS:

Calorie: 229
Carbohydrate: 16g
Fat: 10g
Protein: 15g
Fiber: 1.8g

Prep. Time: 5-7 minutes
Serves: 2

INGREDIENTS:

- 10 pieces spring roll wrappers, separated, quartered
- ¼ pound sharp cheddar cheese, reduced fat, sliced into 2" x ½" matchsticks
- Oil for spraying

INSTRUCTIONS:

1. Preheat the Air Fryer to 400 degrees F.
2. Place cheese matchstick at widest end of quartered spring roll wrapper. Moisten edges and tip of wrapper with water. Fold spring roll wrapper over cheese, and tuck in both ends. Roll spring roll tightly up to the tip. Place this into a freezer-safe container lined with saran wrap. Repeat step for all cheese and spring roll wrappers.
3. Freeze for an hour before frying.
4. Spray small amount of oil all over cheese matchsticks. Place a generous handful inside Air Fryer basket. Fry for 3 to 5 minutes, or only until wrappers turn golden brown. Shake contents of basket once midway through.
5. Remove from basket. Set on plates. Repeat step for remaining breaded cheese sticks. Serve.

ZUCCHINI CRISPS

NUTRITION FACTS:

Calorie: 15.2

Carbohydrate: 3.6g

Fat: 0.1g

Protein: 0.6g

Fiber: 1.3g

Prep. Time: 1 hour

Serves: 2

INGREDIENTS:

- 2 zucchini, sliced into ⅛-inch thick disk
- pinch of sea salt
- white pepper to taste
- olive oil for drizzling

INSTRUCTIONS:

1. Preheat the Air Fryer to 330 degrees F.
2. Put zucchini in a bowl with salt. Let sit in a colander to drain for 30 minutes.
3. Layer zucchini in a baking dish. Drizzle in oil. Season with pepper. Place baking dish in the Air fryer basket. Cook for 30 minutes.
4. Adjust seasoning. Serve.

TORTILLAS IN GREEN MANGO SALSA

NUTRITION FACTS:

Calorie: 128

Carbohydrate: 8.6g

Fat: 3.6g

Protein: 2.7g

Fiber: 5.7g

Prep. Time: 30 minutes

Serves: 4

INGREDIENTS:

Tortillas

- 4 pieces corn tortillas
- 1 Tbsp. olive oil
- 1/16 tsp. sea salt

GREEN MANGO SALSA

- 1 green/unripe mango, minced
- 1 red/ripe Roma tomato, preferably, minced
- 1 shallot, peeled, minced
- 1 fresh jalapeno pepper, minced
- ¼ red bell pepper, minced
- 4 Tbsp. fresh cilantro, minced
- ¼ cup lime juice, freshly squeezed
- 1/16 tsp. salt

INSTRUCTIONS:

1. Preheat the Air Fryer to 400 degrees F.
2. Mix lime juice and salt in a bowl. Stir until solids dissolve. Add in remaining salsa ingredients. Chill in fridge for at least 30 minutes. Stir again just before using.
3. Lightly brush oil on both sides of tortillas. Cut these into large triangles.
4. Place generous handful of sliced tortillas in the Air Fryer basket. Fry these for 10 minutes or until bread blisters and turns golden brown. Shake contents of basket once midway

through.

5. Place cooked pieces on a plate. Repeat step for remaining tortillas. Season with salt.

6. Place equal portions of crispy tortillas on plates. Serve with green mango and tomato salsa on the side.

SQUID IN MAYO DIP

NUTRITION FACTS:

Calorie: 100

Carbohydrate: 10.6g

Fat: 7.12g

Protein: 14.43g

Fiber: 1.9g

Prep. Time: 33-35 minutes

Serves: 4

SQUID AND MARINADE

- 1½ pounds frozen squid rings, thawed
- 1 tsp. cayenne powder
- 1 cup, 8 oz. plain yogurt
- Dash of red pepper flakes
- Pinch of sea salt

BREADING

- 2 eggs, whisked
- 2 cups almond flour, finely milled
- 2 cups almond meal, coarse milled

MAYO

- 1 Tbsp. mayonnaise
- ½ cup sour cream
- 2 Tbsp. lemon juice, fresh-squeezed
- 1 sprig, largefresh cilantro, minced
- Pinch of sea salt
- Pinch of white pepper to taste

INSTRUCTIONS:

1. Preheat the Air Fryer to 330 degrees F.
2. Mix mayonnaise, sour cream, lemon juice, cilantro, salt, and pepper in a bowl. Set aside.
3. In another bowl, combine squid, cayenne powder, yogurt, red pepper flakes, and salt. Chill for 30 minutes. Drain.
4. Combine marinade and eggs. Whisk well. Dredge quid in almond flour, then egg mixture, then almond meal.
5. Layer squid inside the Air fryer basket and fry for 3 minutes or until golden brown.
6. Drain on paper towels. Serve with lemony-mayo dip.

AIR FRIED CARROTS AND PARSNIPS

NUTRITION FACTS:

Calorie: 163
Carbohydrate: 34.2g
Fat: 2.9g
Protein: 2.8
Fiber: 7.8g

Prep. Time: 7-10 minutes
Serves: 4

FRIED CARROTS AND PARSNIPS

- 2 large carrots, sliced into thick matchsticks
- 2 large parsnips, sliced into thick matchsticks
- 1½ cups almond flour, finely milled
- 2 large eggs, whisked
- 1½ cups almond meal
- Pinch of sea salt
- Pinch of cinnamon powder, to taste

DIRECTIONS:

1. Preheat the Air Fryer to 330 degrees F.
2. Dredge fruit in almond flour first, and then into eggs, and into almond meal; shake off excess starch. Carefully slide breaded pieces into the Air fryer basket.
3. Fry until crisp and golden, flipping often. Drain on paper towels. Season with sea salt; serve.

BLUEBERRY MUFFINS

NUTRITION FACTS:

Calorie: 277

Carbohydrate: 28g

Fat: 16g

Protein: 4.5g

Fiber: 1g

Prep. Time: 15-20 minutes

Serves: 4

INGREDIENTS:

- 2 Tbsp. almond flour
- 1 cup fresh blueberries, rinsed well, drained
- 1 tsp. brown sugar

DRY INGREDIENTS

- 2 Tbsp. almond flour
- 2 tsp. baking powder
- ½ tsp. salt
- 1½ cups cake flour, sifted twice
- ½ cup stevia

WET INGREDIENTS

- 1 egg, whisked until frothy
- 2 tsp. vanilla extract
- 1 cup Greek yogurt
- 1/3 cup coconut oil, melted

INSTRUCTIONS:

1. Preheat the Air Fryer to 355 degrees F.
2. Using a pastry brush, lightly grease four 4 oz. disposable aluminum muffin tins.
3. Place blueberries and flour in a bowl. Toss so that blueberries are well coated.
4. Mix dry ingredients in a bowl, and dry ingredients in another.

5. Pour wet ingredients into the dry ones. Mix until just combined. Fold in floured blueberries.

6. Place equal portions into prepared muffin tins. Sprinkle equal portions of brown sugar on top of each.

7. Place muffin tins in one layer into Air Fryer basket. Cook these for 10 minutes, or until toothpick inserted in the center comes out clean. Turn off heat, but keep muffins in the basket for another 5 minutes. Remove from basket.

8. Serve warm.

AIR FRIED RIPE PLANTAINS

NUTRITION FACTS:

Calorie: 209

Carbohydrate: 29g

Fat: 8g

Protein: 2.9g

Fiber: 3.5g

Prep. Time: 10 minutes

Serves: 2

INGREDIENTS

- 2 pieces large ripe plantain, peeled, sliced into inch thick disks
- 1 Tbsp. coconut butter, unsweetened

INSTRUCTIONS:

- Preheat the Air Fryer to 350°F.
- Brush small amount of coconut butter on all sides of plantain disks.
- Place one even layer into Air Fryer basket, making sure none overlap or touch. Fry plantains for 10 minutes.
- Remove from basket. Place on plates. Repeat step for all plantains.
- While plantains are still warm. Serve.

GARLIC BREAD WITH CHEESE DIP

NUTRITION FACTS:

Calorie: 209
Carbohydrate: 29g
Fat: 8g
Protein: 2.9g
Fiber: 3.5g

Prep. Time: 10 minutes
Serves: 8

INGREDIENTS:

Fried garlic bread

- 1 medium baguette, halved lengthwise, cut sides toasted
- 2 garlic cloves, whole
- 4 Tbsp. extra virgin olive oil
- 2 Tbsp. fresh parsley, minced

BLUE CHEESE DIP

- 1 Tbsp. fresh parsley, minced
- ¼ cup fresh chives, minced
- ¼ tsp. Tabasco sauce
- 1 Tbsp. lemon juice, freshly squeezed
- ½ cup Greek yogurt, low fat
- ¼ cup blue cheese, reduced fat
- 1/16 tsp. salt
- 1/16 tsp. white pepper

INSTRUCTIONS:

1. Preheat machine to 400 degrees F.
2. Combine oil and parsley in a small bowl.
3. Vigorously rub garlic cloves on cut/toasted sides of baguette. Dispose garlic nubs.
4. Using a pastry brush, spread parsley-infused oil on cut side of bread.
5. Place bread cut-side down on a chopping board. Slice into inch-thick half-moons.

6. Place bread slices in Air Fryer basket. Fry for 3 to 5 minutes or until bread browns a little. Shake contents of basket once midway through. Place cooked pieces on a serving platter. Repeat step for remaining bread.

7. To prepare blue cheese dip: mix ingredients in a bowl.

8. Place equal portions of fried bread on plates. Serve with blue cheese dip on the side.

FRIED MIXED VEGGIES WITH AVOCADO DIP

NUTRITION FACTS:

Calorie: 109

   Carbohydrate: 4.0g

   Fat: 2.6g

   Protein: 2.9g

   Fiber: 2.5g

   Prep. Time: 10 minutes

   Serves: 4

INGREDIENTS

- Oil for spraying

AVOCADO-FETA DIP

- 1 avocado, pitted, peeled, flesh scooped out
- 4 oz. feta cheese, reduced fat
- 2 leeks, minced
- 1 lime, freshly squeezed
- ¼ cup fresh parsley, chopped roughly
- 1/16 tsp. black pepper
- 1/16 tsp. salt

VEGETABLES

- 1 zucchini, sliced into matchsticks
- 1 carrot, sliced into matchsticks
- 1 cup panko breadcrumbs, add more if needed
- 1 parsnip, sliced into matchsticks
- 1 large egg, whisked, add more if needed
- 1 cup all-purpose flour, add more if needed
- ⅛ tsp. flaky sea salt

INSTRUCTIONS:

1. Preheat the Air Fryer to 400 degrees F.
2. Season carrots, parsnips and zucchini with salt.
3. Dredge carrots into flour first, then egg, and finally into breadcrumbs. Place breaded pieces on a baking sheet lined with parchment paper. Repeat step for all carrots. Then do the same for parsnips and zucchini.
4. Lightly spray vegetables with oil. Place generous handful of carrots in the Air Fryer basket. Fry for 10 minutes or until breading turns golden brown, shaking contents of the basket once midway. Place cooked pieces on a plate. Repeat step for remaining carrots.
5. Do previous step for parsnips, and then zucchini.
6. For the dip, except for salt, place remaining ingredients in a food processor. Pulse a couple of times, and then process to desired consistency scraping down sides of machine often. Taste. Add salt only if needed. Place in airtight container. Chill until needed.
7. Place equal portions of cooked vegetables on plates. Serve with small amount of avocado-feta dip on the side.

SWEET POTATO CRISPS

NUTRITION FACTS:

Calorie: 122
Carbohydrate: 15g
Fat: 6g
Protein: 1g
Fiber: 0g

Prep. Time: 10 minutes
Serves: 8

INGREDIENTS:

- 2 large sweet potatoes, shaved thin using mandolin
- Spanish paprika and sea salt to taste

DIPS, OPTIONAL

- ¼ cup cashew cheese
- ¼ cup spinach walnut pesto

INSTRUCTIONS:

1. Preheat Air Fryer to 330 degrees F.
2. Place sweet potatoes flat on baking sheets with spaces in between pieces. Drizzle in oil; season lightly with paprika and sea salt.
3. Put baking sheet inside the Air fryer basket. Fry for 30 minutes. Cool completely to room temperature before serving. Serve with cashew cheese and spinach walnut pesto.

AIR FRIED PLANTAINS IN COCONUT SAUCE

NUTRITION FACTS:

Calorie: 236

Carbohydrate: 0g

Fat: 1.5g

Protein: 1g

Fiber: 1.8g

Prep. Time: 10 minutes

Serves: 8

INGREDIENTS:

- 6 ripe plantains, peeled, quartered lengthwise
- 1 can coconut cream
- 1 Tbsp. Splenda

INSTRUCTIONS:

1. Preheat the Air Fryer to 330 degrees F.
2. Pour coconut cream in thick-bottomed saucepan set over high heat; bring to boil. Reduce heat to lowest setting; simmer uncovered until cream is reduced by half and darkens in color. Turn off heat.
3. Whisk in honey until smooth. Cool completely before using. Lightly grease non-stick skillet with coconut oil.
4. Layer plantains in the Air fryer basket and fry until golden on both sides; drain on paper towels. Place plantain into plates.
5. Drizzle in small amount of coconut sauce. Serve.

APPLE CINNAMON PASTRY

NUTRITION FACTS:

Calorie: 74

Carbohydrate: 13g

Fat: 2g

Protein: 0g

Fiber: 0g

Prep. Time: 10-15 minutes

Serves: 4

INGREDIENTS:

- 100 grams puff pastry, sliced into squares
- 2 Tbsp. whole milk
- Water for sealing

FILLING

- ½ cup apples, minced
- 1/16 tsp. quick cooking oats
- ⅛ tsp. cinnamon powder
- 1/16 tsp. butter, unsalted

INSTRUCTIONS:

- Preheat the Air Fryer to 400°F. Place puff pastry on a baking sheet lined with parchment paper.
- Combine filling ingredients in a bowl. Divide into eight equal portions.
- Place one filling portion into prepared puff pastry.
- Moisten edges of pastry with water. Fold these over into a triangle to seal. Using tines of a fork, press down on the edges.
- Brush small amount of milk on top of puff pastries.
- Place these in an even layer into Air Fryer basket, making sure none overlap. Fry for 10 minutes, or until pastries brown. Remove from basket.
- Serve equal portions.

CONCLUSION

Thank you again for purchasing this book!

I hope this book was able to help you understand how you can overcome the onset of diabetes through food choices. The beauty of this cookbook is that it is a one-two punch of weight loss and blood sugar control.

The next step is to try the recipes or make variations of your own. What is important is that you are now more aware of the kind of food that you allowed and not allowed to eat. If you have favorite food and would still like a taste of them, you may come up with your own healthy and low carb version. All you have to do is substitute all ingredients to reduced fat, low carb, and nonfat. Remember to keep track of your meals to see how well you have progressed.

Finally, if you enjoyed this book, please take the time to share your thoughts and post a review on Amazon. It'd be greatly appreciated!

Thank you and good luck!